How Much Sugar is Too Much?

MANAGING DIABETES

Dr Yatish Agarwal
Rekha Agarwal

जय विज्ञान JAI VIGYAN
2004
वैज्ञानिक जागरूकता वर्ष
Year of Scientific Awareness

Rajkamal

Rajkamal Books
1-B Netaji Subhash Marg
Daryaganj, New Delhi – 110 002
Tel: 011-232 74463; 232 88769 *Fax*: 23278144
E-mail: Info@rajkamalprakashan.com

ISBN: 978-81-267-1043-0

First published in the *Year of Scientific Awareness*, 2004

This edition, 2012

Advisors

Dr Umesh Kansara
Chief of Diabetic Clinic
VM Medical College &
Safdarjung Hospital, New Delhi

Dr. Ashok Damir
Chief Diabetologist
Delhi Diabetes Centre
New Delhi

Editor : Manju Gupta
Creative Director : Abhimanyu Sinha
Graphics : Tapas Sarkar, Naresh Sharma
Production : Mahesh Chandra

The authors can be reached on the e-mail at: **dryatish@yahoo.com**

₹ 60

Printed at B.K. Offset
Shahadra, Delhi-110 032

This book is intended not as a substitute for personal medical advice but as a supplement to that advice for the patient who wishes to understand more about his or her condition. Before taking any form of treatment, you must always consult your physician. You should note that advances in medical science occur rapidly and some of the information about drugs and treatment contained in this book may soon be out of date.

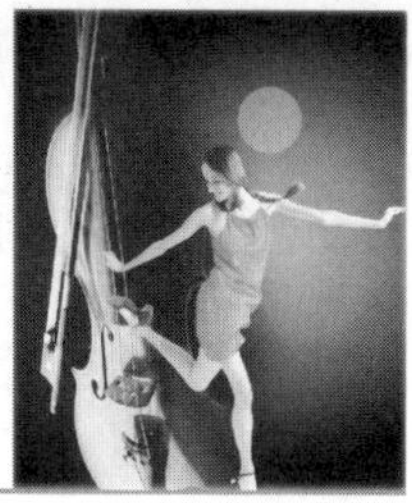

Contents

How Much of Sugar is Too Much
Understanding Diabetes

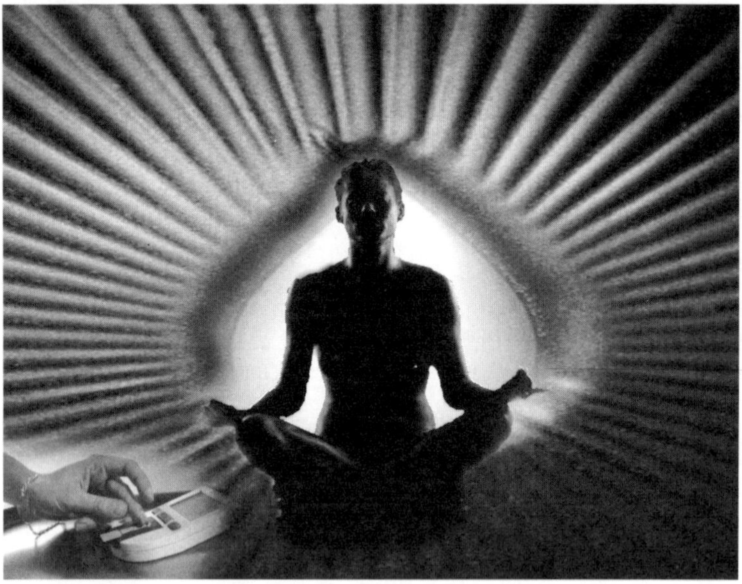

Diabetes is a malady recognized since the ancient times. Named *madhumeha* by the *ayurvedacharyas* in the Sanskrit era, it today affects millions of people worldwide. Due to changed living habits, its numbers have burgeoned in the past few decades.

Until a few years ago, diabetes was a disease mostly of the affluent world. This has now changed. Emergent societies are also now caught in its web. Life there too has lost out to the forces of mechanization, changed eating habits, crammed routines, and modern-day stresses and strains.

O health! Health! The blessing of the rich! The riches of the poor! Who can buy thee at too dear a rate, since there is no enjoying this world without thee?

Ben Jonson
Volpone

Today, more than 150 million people are affected by diabetes across the globe. This number is likely to cross the 300 million mark by 2025. The situation is most grim in the third world countries, where the number of cases is set to rise by a galloping 170 per cent.

Projected numbers of people with diabetes in 2025

India	57,243,000	Brazil	11,603,000
China	37,555,000	Indonesia	12,427,000
US	21,892,000	Pakistan	14,523,000
Russia	12,240,000	Mexico	11,684,000
Japan	8,543,000	Egypt	8,802,000

The forecast for India is most severe. Unless speedy preventive steps are taken, more than 57 million of her people will have diabetes by 2025. This shall make India the number one hub of diabetes in the world. The past few years have witnessed a major rise in the number of cases. Today, roughly 10-12 per cent adults in urban India, and 3-4 per cent in countryside suffer from diabetes. Unfortunately, more than one-half do not even know about their disease. The reason: There are often no definite symptoms to warn you that it exists.

Diabetes can occur at any age. It affects men and women equally. Community studies have found that the disease makes its foray at an earlier age in India than in many other parts of the world. Roughly 38 per cent people with diabetes were found to be younger than 40, and roughly 5 per cent were less than 25 years of age.

Diabetes also runs in families. If an immediate family member—father, mother, sister or brother—has diabetes, your risk goes up considerably. Perhaps due to this reason, its prevalence is higher among those communities, where marriages within the family are a routine or the size of the community is small.

What is diabetes?

Diabetes is a disorder of your metabolism—the way your body uses digested food to fuel the activities of its billions of cells. Normally, your digestive system cleaves carbohydrates—the sugary, starchy portion of the food you eat—into a sugar called glucose. Glucose then enters your bloodstream, ready to energize your cells.

So that your cells can take in the delivery of glucose, insulin, a hormone produced by your pancreas, must 'escort' it in. Normally, your pancreas works all the time. Tucked deep inside the abdomen, this 3-ounce gland keeps a tab on the amount of glucose in your blood. When it senses a rise, such as after a meal, it becomes more active. The secretion of insulin increases, and it escorts glucose from your bloodstream to your individual cells. As glucose enters your cells, its amount in the blood drops, and it soon returns to the basal level.

Mother Nature has also given you a storehouse for excess glucose. It is the liver, which can keep glucose tucked away in the form of glycogen. Again, insulin is the password to escort the glucose into this 'cupboard'.

A host of other hormones also play a role in this intricate metabolism. Glucagon, growth hormone, cortisol and epinephrine—all work in the reverse manner. They push up the amount of glucose in the blood under certain stressful situations, when the body's energy demand suddenly rises.

This wonderful mechanism is watchful of the body's needs at all times, but it is clever enough to maintain your blood glucose level within a narrow normal range. The process, however, is disrupted when diabetes strikes. A deficit of insulin occurs, or it loses its effect. Glucose enters into the cells only in limited amounts. Some of the glucose then builds up in your blood, overflows into your urine and passes from your body unused. The ancients were wise to this, and therefore, they named the disease, *madhumeha*, or sweet urine. The modern term, *diabetes mellitus*, means much the same.

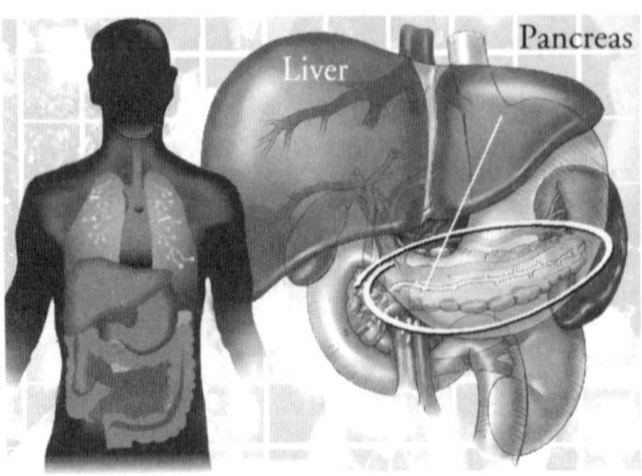

Types of diabetes

Diabetes can occur in a variety of situations, and probably each deserves a different name, but broadly, the disease has four major categories.

Type 1

Type 1 diabetes usually arises in childhood or teen years. Symptoms generally appear suddenly, and when the diagnosis is made, the parents and child often react with disbelief and shock. The disease occurs due to the destruction of insulin-producing units in the pancreas. The body is no longer able to produce insulin, and life is possible only with the help of daily injections of the hormone.

Viewed as an autoimmune disease, it occurs because the body's immune system goes haywire, and attacks and destroys the insulin-producing cells, known as beta cells, in the pancreas. Genetic and environmental factors work hand in glove to fool the immune system in to producing antibodies against the pancreas cells.

Researchers have identified several possible genes and a number of viruses that may play a role in causation of type 1 diabetes, but the exact mechanism is still under investigation. The disease accounts for roughly 5 per cent of all diabetes cases.

Type 2

Roughly 95-96 per cent people with diabetes have type 2 disease. Formerly, it was thought to be a disease which commenced in middle age, but that's not the case any more. Even children and teens now have type 2 diabetes, and the number is growing.

In this form of diabetes, either the cells stop responding to insulin or the pancreas produces it in short supply. As a result, the body's fine act of regulating the glucose level in the blood goes awry.

A number of genes probably work backstage to cause the disease. In addition, the disease has a strong relationship with obesity. About 80 per cent of people with this form of the disease are significantly overweight.

Symptoms in type 2 diabetes often develop slowly. Hence, you may not immediately recognize that you are sick.

Gestational diabetes

Gestational diabetes is an ephemeral condition associated with pregnancy. In this situation, blood glucose levels increase during pregnancy but usually return to normal after delivery. This happens in about 2-5 per cent of pregnant women.

Gestational diabetes typically develops during the second half of pregnancy—especially in the third trimester—and usually goes away after the baby is born. But more than half of all women who experience gestational diabetes develop type 2 diabetes later in life.

If you develop gestational diabetes, being aware of your condition and controlling your blood sugar level throughout the remainder of your pregnancy can reduce complications in you and your baby.

Secondary to other conditions

Diabetes mellitus may also develop as a secondary condition linked to another illnesses or to medications that can interfere with the production of insulin or its action. Approximately 1 per cent of all diagnosed cases of diabetes fall under this group. Inflammation of the pancreas (pancreatitis), adrenal or pituitary gland disorders, myotonic dystrophy (a genetic syndrome), or medications, such as corticosteroids, may lead to a persistent rise in blood sugar.

Symptoms

Many people are unaware that they have diabetes. That's because there are often no early symptoms to recognize the type 2 disease. When symptoms do develop from persistently high blood glucose, they vary, but often the diagnosis is made because of an indirect sign or a blood test. However, sometimes people also report the classic symptoms given below:

Excessive thirst and increased urination. When you have high levels of glucose in your blood, your kidneys cannot reabsorb all of the filtered sugar. The circulating sugar carries water with it, and this leads to more frequent urination. Since this draws out water from your tissues, you feel an excessive thirst.

Constant fatigue and weakness. Glucose is your body's main fuel. When you have diabetes, it doesn't get to your cells, and this makes you feel constantly tired, exhausted and weak.

Unexplained weight loss or gain. As your body struggles to make up for the constant loss of glucose, you may eat more than usual and gain weight. In other people, the opposite occurs: you lose weight even though you're eating more. This is especially true if you have type 1 diabetes.

Slow healing cuts or bruises. Excess amount of glucose in the blood plays havoc with the natural healing mechanism of body tissues, and there is an increased tendency to infection.

Frequent skin, urinary and genital infections. Diabetes blocks your body's natural healing process and its ability to fight off infections. For women, bladder and vaginal infections are especially common. Boils may also occur very frequently in both sexes. The skin may also become dry and itchy.

Pyorrhoea and loss of teeth. High levels of blood glucose may weaken your mouth's ability to fight germs, increasing the risk of infection in the gums and the jawbone. This may cause foul breath, pyorrhoea, pockets of pus in your gums, pulling away of gums from your teeth, and loosened teeth. In fact, many times the disease is brought to attention because of these changes.

Numbness and tingling in feet and hands. Long-standing diabetes can damage your nerves, and this can produce a number of symptoms. The most common symptom is a tingling feeling and a loss of sensation that occurs mainly in your feet and hands. You may also feel a burning pain in your legs, feet, arms and hands. Damage to the nerves that control digestion can lead to nausea, diarrhoea or constipation. In men, diabetes can cause impotence due to damage to the nerve that facilitates erection.

Blurred vision. Excess glucose in your blood affects the hydration of the natural lenses in your eyes, and this can affect their ability to focus. But once the sugar is under control, your vision will improve in time.

Prolonged diabetes can cause the formation of tiny frail blood vessels in your eyes that can bleed. The blood vessels themselves do not produce symptoms, but bleeding from the vessels can cause dark spots, and sometimes, blindness.

Other signs. If neglected, persistent high levels of glucose in your blood can cause damage to your body's small and large blood vessels. This is the root of several complications. You are liable to develop kidney failure, heart disease, and stroke, unless you are watchful. Keeping your blood glucose under control is the best guarantee against damage.

Diagnosing diabetes

The amount of sugar in your blood is the best indicator of the disease. It does naturally fluctuate, but within a narrow range. Following an overnight (at least for eight hours) fast, most people normally have blood glucose levels between 70-109 mg/dl. However, if your fasting blood glucose rises to a consistent 126 mg/dl or more, it is indicative of diabetes. Levels between 110 and 125 mg/dl are pre-diabetic and indicate that you must be watchful. It is a sign that

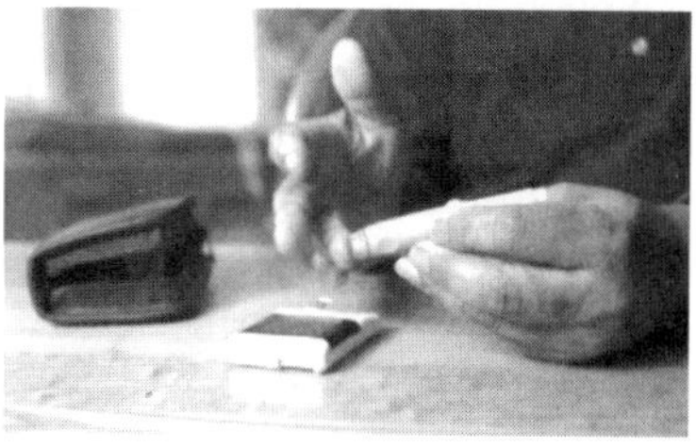

you are at a high risk of developing the disease.

Since an undiagnosed disease carries a risk of serious complications, the best safeguard is to undertake a fasting and after-breakfast blood glucose test at least once every three years. This safeguard is necessary once you are 45. If you are overweight, remain habitually physically inactive, have a first-degree relative who has diabetes, have abnormally high blood cholesterol and triglyceride levels, suffer from high blood pressure, or your blood glucose has been more than 110 mg/dl before, then you should take the test more often. Women who have polycystic ovarian disease, or have had a baby of more than 9 pounds birthweight, or have been diagnosed with gestational diabetes, should also be more vigilant.

A casual blood glucose level of 200 mg/dl or more is also indicative of the disease. However, to confirm the diagnosis, you may be asked to take the oral glucose tolerance test. A fasting blood glucose level of 126 mg/dl or more, and a post-glucose two-hour blood glucose level of 200 mg/dl or more corroborates the diagnosis of diabetes.

Managing the disease

Exercise, diet, reduction in weight, self-care and medication are the five integral components of managing diabetes. Good control over blood sugar is key to avoiding complications. If you succeed in this mission, you could enjoy a normal life. On the other hand, if you are careless about the disease, the risk of complications rockets. Not only you could suffer a premature death, you may experience a crippling blow and suffer a serious deterioration in the quality of life because of blinding complications in the eye, kidney damage, coronary heart disease, stroke or neuropathy.

If you have type 1 diabetes, the treatment is straightforward. You must take insulin by injection each day. The number of daily injections prescribed depend on your individual needs.

If you have type 2 diabetes and have trouble controlling your blood sugar with diet and exercise alone, you would be prescribed one of several oral medications. These medications can help your pancreas produce more insulin or help insulin to work better in your body. If your blood sugar is too high, or oral medications do not work well, you might have to rely on insulin injections for a while. Once things improve, you could return to oral medication.

As it is a disease that lasts, you must treat diabetes for life. From time to time, you might feel tempted to stop your regular treatment and try out the products which promise a cure and are sold through billboards and advertisements. People may also tell you about miraculous cures worked by alternative systems of medicine. You may try them, if you like, but be rational. Check them out on the basis of sound scientific reason, and if a cure still appeals to you, you may consider it, but do not be negligent about blood sugar level during this period.

There are definite goals that you should try and achieve while to rein in the disease. Let's take a look at them:

Living with diabetes: goals to meet

Control your blood sugar	
Fasting blood glucose	90-130 mg/dl
Two-hours after a meal	180 mg/dl
Glycosylated haemoglobin (HbA_1C)	less than 7 per cent
Control your blood pressure	
Maintain blood pressure	lower than 130/80 mm Hg
Control your weight	
Reduce your weight	bring your body mass index to 24 or less
Control your lipid numbers	
LDL cholesterol	less than 100 mg/dl
Triglyceride	less than 150 mg/dl
HDL cholesterol	over 40 mg/dl

Diabetes is a serious illness, but it can be controlled. If you are willing to do your part, you can continue to enjoy an active and healthy life. The road to good health begins here!

Living Well

Prevention the Best Medicine

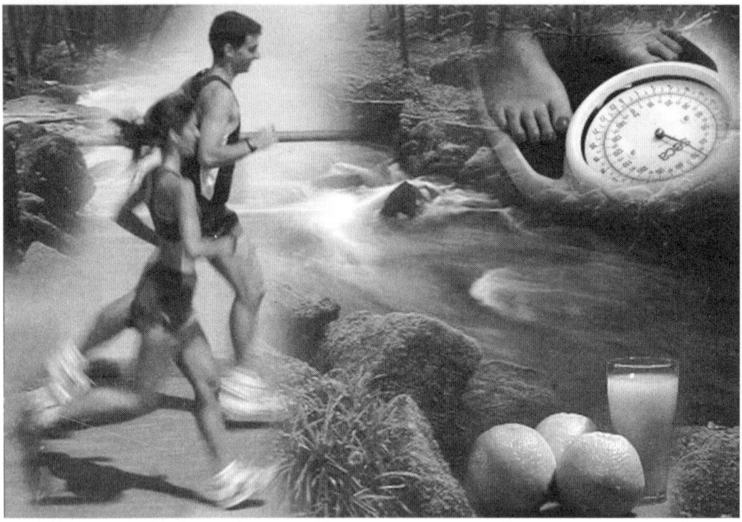

More than 95 per cent of the people with diabetes suffer from type 2 disease. Since the illness can jeopardize life, and carries a high risk of serious complications, efforts are afoot to find the risk factors that lead to development of the disease. During the last one decade, large community studies have identified the culprits, and on that basis, preventive strategies have been put together. Let's see how:

Factors that increase your risk

Despite what people believe, diabetes is not caused by eating too much sugar. Even though some of its secrets may still elude us, recent research has confirmed the lifestyle factors and health

The preservation of health is a duty. Few seem conscious that there is such a thing as physical morality.

Herbert Spencer
Education

conditions that increase the risk for diabetes.

Family history. You are more likely to develop diabetes if someone in your immediate family—your father, mother, brother or sister has the disease. This genetic association manifests most strongly if your sibling suffers from diabetes. The risk also goes up considerably if both your parents have diabetes.

Weight. Being overweight is by far the greatest risk factor for type 2 diabetes. More than 80 per cent of people who develop the disease are overweight. The more fat you have, the more resistant your cells become to your own insulin. Studies show that the risk for developing type 2 diabetes increases by 4 per cent for every pound of excess weight a person carries. It is as though the fat blocks insulin from doing its job.

Physical inactivity. Individuals who lead a totally sedentary life run a big risk of developing diabetes. Their cells become resistant to insulin, and this causes a rise in blood sugar.

Blood pressure and cholesterol link. If your blood pressure is persistently over 140/90 mm Hg, serum triglyceride levels are greater than 250 mg/dl, and HDL cholesterol is less than 35 mg/dl, than it's time to pull up your socks. These parameters indicate a high risk of developing diabetes.

Womanly risks. A woman who has suffered from polycystic ovarian disease, or a diabetes while she was pregnant, or had given birth to a baby who was more than 9 pounds at birth should always be on the vigil for diabetes.

Age. As you grow older, your risk of type 2 diabetes increases. The risk grows once you go past the age of 45, but even younger people in the twenties, thirties and early forties must be careful. Type 2 diabetes is increasingly being diagnosed in young people.

The obesity connection

Your weight and your risk for developing diabetes are closely related. If you feel concerned, check your body mass index, or measure your waist, to know how much weight you have.

Body mass index

Body mass index (BMI) is a measurement based on a formula that takes into account your weight and your height in determining how much fat you carry around your body.

To determine your BMI, locate your height on the chart given on the next page and follow that row across until you reach the column with the weight nearest yours. Look at the top of that column for the corresponding BMI rating. A BMI of 19 to 24 is considered healthy. A BMI of 25 to 29 signifies being overweight, and a BMI of 30 or more indicates obesity. As you go over 24, your risk of developing diabetes goes up.

Body mass index

	Healthy		*Overweight*		*Obesity*				
BMI →	19	24	25	29	30	35	40	45	50
Height (*Feet & inches*)	*Weight (in kilograms)*								
4'10"	41	52	54	63	65	75	87	98	108
4'10"	41	52	54	63	65	75	87	98	108
4'11"	43	54	56	65	67	79	90	101	112
5'0"	44	56	58	67	70	81	93	105	116
5'1"	45	58	60	70	72	84	96	108	120
5'2"	47	60	62	72	75	97	99	112	124
5'3"	49	62	64	74	77	90	102	115	128
5'4"	50	64	66	77	79	93	105	119	132
5'5"	52	65	68	79	82	95	109	123	136
5'6"	54	67	70	81	85	98	112	126	140
5'7"	55	70	72	84	87	101	116	130	145
5'8"	57	72	75	86	90	105	119	134	149
5'9"	58	74	77	89	92	107	123	138	154
5'10"	60	76	79	92	95	110	126	142	158
5'11"	62	78	81	95	98	114	130	146	163
6'0"	64	80	84	97	100	117	134	150	167
6'1"	65	81	86	100	103	120	137	155	172
6'2"	67	85	88	102	106	124	147	159	177

Waist circumference

Extra weight is bad enough, but it also matters where the weight is stored. If you carry most of the weight around your belly, you are 'apple-shaped'. If it is around your hips and thighs, you are 'pear-shaped'. Where you store weight is for the most part inherited from your parents, but, if you are apple-shaped, you are at a greater risk for heart disease, diabetes and high blood pressure. In any case, if you carry too much weight, you should take steps to lose the extra fat.

To determine whether you are carrying too much weight around your belly, measure your waist circumference. Find the highest point on each of your hipbones and measure across your abdomen just above those highest points. A measurement of more than 39 inches in men and 34 inches in women signifies increased health risks.

Taking steps to prevent diabetes

You may greatly reduce your risk of developing diabetes if you take pre-emptive steps and adopt healthful changes in your living habits. No age is too early, and the sooner you realize the benefits of good nutrition, physical activity, and restriction of weight, the better are your chances of progressing in life without being affected by diabetes. If you are careful, the risk of the disease can be reduced by 50-60 per cent.

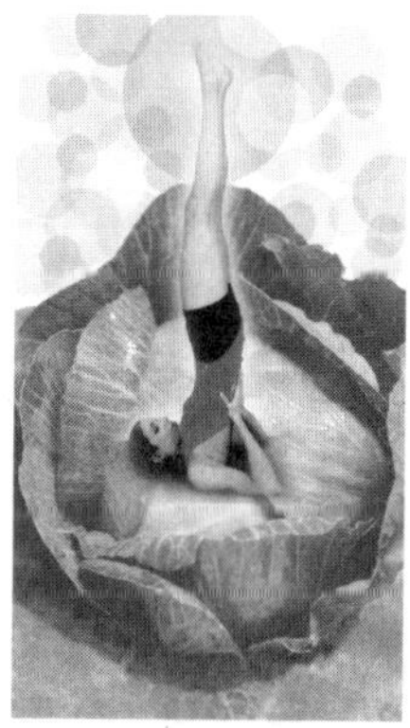

Eat healthy. Restrict your daily calories to suit your weight and lifestyle. Take more fibre, restrict fat to less than 30 per cent of daily calories, and reduce saturated fat intake to less than 10 per cent calories. The less processed food you take, and the more natural food you take, the better it is.

Get moving. Exercise regularly. Take a 30-minute brisk walk most days of the week. If you find it dull, you can swim, cycle, do aerobic dancing or play a sport such as badminton or tennis. The goal should be to do at least 150 minutes of moderately intense physical activity every week.

Maintain a healthy weight. Watch your weight. If your BMI is 24 or over, you must take active measures to lose weight. In 95 per cent cases, the reason for obesity is straightforward: too many calories, and too little activity. Reverse this, and you may profit.

reason. Most sweets have little nutritional value, and just cram your body with unhealthy calories. You can do much better by eating fruits, vegetables, and grain products. The message is simple: do not be paranoid about sweet foods, but do not go overboard either!

In a wholesome diet, carbohydrates should make 50-60 per cent of the daily calories. To plan your meal, you can divide them into four groups: starches, vegetables, fruits and dairy products. Depending on your daily calorie allowance, you can have six or more servings of starches (rice, wheat, beans, potatoes), three to five servings of vegetables, two to four servings of fruit, and two to three servings of dairy food. Natural foods, particularly with a high-fibre content, should be your favourite as they help lower both blood sugar and blood cholesterol.

Proteins

Coined from a Greek word, which means 'of the first importance', proteins are foods essential for the growth and repair of body tissue. They also model haemoglobin, enzymes, chemical messengers, globulin, and albumin, each of which performs an important function in the body.

A normal diet should include 10-20 per cent of the daily calories from protein. In real terms, this means two or three protein servings each day. The best plant sources of protein include legumes — beans, dried peas and lentils; soya products, grains, and peanut butter. Animal foods, including milk, cheese, eggs, meat, fish, and poultry also have high protein content, but are not preferred because of their high-fat content.

Fats

Fats are essential for the body. They provide energy are an integral component of hormones, membranes, and nerve insulation material, and assist in the absorption of fat-soluble vitamins. On the basis of their chemical structure, they are classified into saturated, polyunsaturated, or monounsaturated type. Vegetable fats—found, for example, in some nuts, olives, and certain vegetable oils—are rich in monounsaturated and polyunsaturated fat. On the other hand, fats found in animal foods, including meat, poultry, cream, butter and lard are of the saturated type.

A normal diet should contain no more than 30 per cent of the daily calories from fats. Since monounsaturated and polyunsaturated fats are far healthier, saturated fats should only make one-third or less of these calories. Using low-fat dairy products, and avoiding fried and junk food can meet this objective.

A healthy eating plan

A healthy eating plan is the cornerstone of diabetes management. Remember to:

Stick to a schedule. Eat no more than three meals and two midday snacks a day. Be consistent in the amount of food you eat and the timing of eating. This will help keep your blood sugar at a consistent level. It is more difficult to control your blood sugar if you eat a big supper one day and a small one the next. Also, the more food you eat at one time, the higher your blood sugar will rise. Eating at regularly spaced intervals—meals spaced four to five hours apart—reduces large variations in blood sugar.

Avoid useless calories. *Mithai,* candy, cookies and other sugars are not forbidden. But because they have little nutritional value, eat them in moderation.

Focus on fibre. Eat a variety of fresh fruits, vegetables, beans and whole-grain foods. They contain less of fat and are good sources of vitamins and minerals.

Count your total calories. Even if surplus calories come from a healthy food, they get converted into fat inside your body. That shoots up your weight, increases LDL cholesterol and triglycerides, and may jack up the blood sugar.

How many calories should you take?

Your daily energy requirements are guided by your body weight and the amount of physical activity you do. The arithmetic is simple. The following chart allows you to pick the 'calorie factor' that applies to you:

Calorie requirement/kilogram body weight

Which category of weight do you fit?	*What kind of lifestyle you lead?*	
	Deskbound life	Moderate activity
Overweight	25	30
Normal for height	30	35
Underweight	35	40

Now, to calculate your daily calorie allowance, simply multiply your body weight by this calorie factor. For example, if you weigh 50 kg, are of normal weight and lead a sedentary life, you shall be needing 50 x 30= 1,500 calories a day. You can draw a suitable diet plan and follow the routine. Some sample charts are given on the next two pages.

1,200-calorie diet menu

Early morning (6 am)

Tea/coffee	1 cup

Breakfast (8 am)

Poha	1 plate
Or veggie sandwich	Cucumber/tomato and 2 slices
Or stuffed *missi roti*	2
Or *namkeen dalia*	3 tablespoons
Fat-free milk	250 ml
Fruit	100 gm

Midday snack (11 am)

Paneer	2 small pieces
Or boiled egg	one
Tea/coffee (no sugar)	1 cup

Lunch (1 pm)

Chappati	2
Or rice	1 cup
Beans (*dal*)/black gram	1 cup
Yoghurt	1 cup
Green vegetables	1 cup
Salad	½ plate

Evening snack (4 pm)

Fruit juice	1 cup

Dinner (8-9 pm)

Mixed vegetable soup	1 bowl
Chappati	2
Lentil/soyabean/beans (*dal*)	1 cup
Vegetable (pumpkin/cabbage/ fresh beans/asparagus/mixed, etc.)	1 cup
Salad	½ plate
Daily allowance of cooking oil	3 tsp

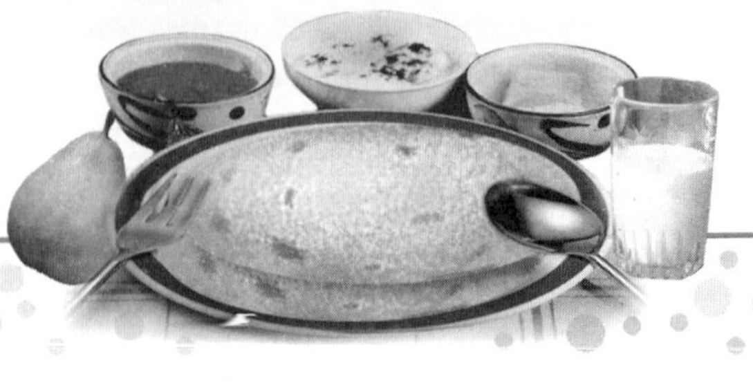

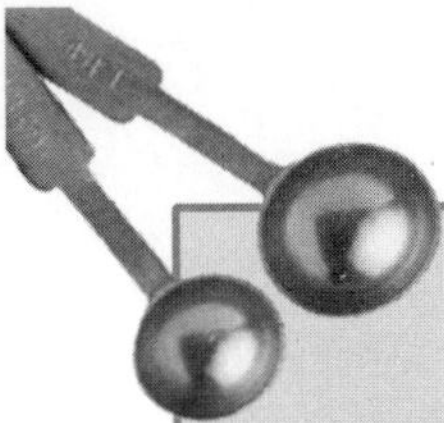
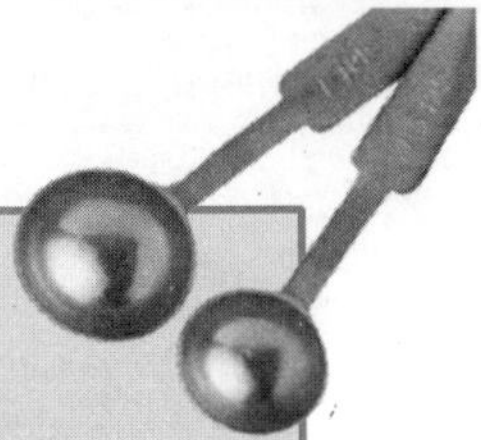

1,500-calorie diet menu

Early morning (6 am)

Tea/coffee	1 cup

Breakfast (8 am)

Bread slices	2
Boiled egg	1
Or milk	200 ml
Tea/coffee	1 cup
Fruit	1

Midday snack (11 am)

Fruit	1

Lunch (1 pm)

Chappati	2
Or rice	1 cup
Dal	1 cup
Green vegetable	1 cup
Yoghurt	½ cup
Tomato /cucumber	1

Evening snack (4 pm)

Tea/coffee	1 cup
Upma	¾ cup

Dinner (8-9 pm)

Chappati	3
Green gram *dal*	1 cup
Or fish/chicken	2 pieces
Vegetable (pumpkin/cabbage/ fresh beans/asparagus/mixed, etc.)	1 cup
Roasted *papad*	1
Tomato/cucumber	1

Bedtime

Milk	1 cup
Daily allowance of cooking oil	4 tsp

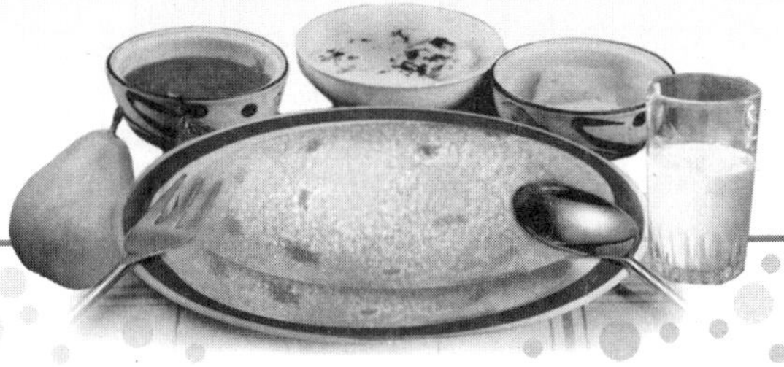

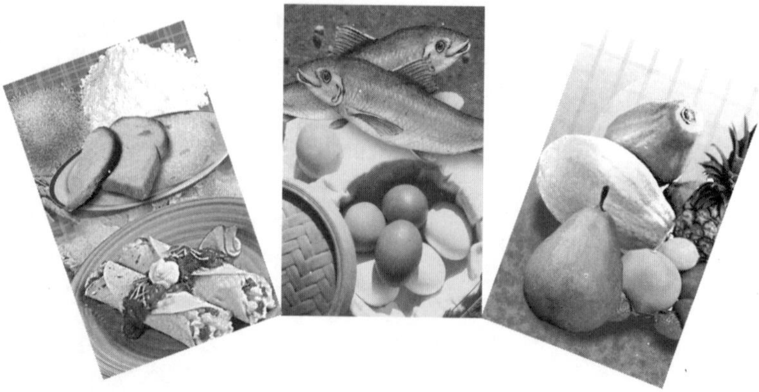

Food exchanges

To break the monotony in your eating plan, you may exchange foods in the diet menu in a variety of ways. Some examples are provided here:

- *One chappati equals:*
  - ½ cup cooked rice
  - 1½ slices of brown bread
  - ¾ cup ready-to-eat cereal
  - 1 medium potato
- *One apple equals:*
  - 2 plums
  - 1 pear
  - 2 oranges
  - 1 guava
  - ¼ papaya
  - ½ cup 100 per cent fruit juice
- *Milk products:*
  - 1cup low-fat milk or
  - 1cup low-fat yoghurt
- *One egg equals:*
  - 200 gm milk
  - 100 gm fish
  - 85 gm skinless poultry or lean meat
  - 65 gm liver
  - ½ cup cooked beans, dried peas or lentils

Role of fenugreek seeds, jamun and bittergourd

Since long, *vaids*, *hakims*, and physicians have tried different foods for their possible blood sugar-lowering properties. Ayurveda recognizes at least three such foods: seeds of fenugreek (*methi*), *jamun* fruit, and the fresh juice of bittergourd (*karela*). Modern-day biochemists and scientists who have been trying to discover novel treatments for diabetes have taken considerable interest in the subject, and have come up with some interesting findings.

The beneficial effect of fenugreek (*methi*) seeds has been borne out by some recent studies. Scientists believe that this good effect relates to the high fibre content and an active alkaloid, trigonelline, found in the fenugreek seeds. Based on this finding, some nutritionists prescribe 25-50 gm fenugreek seeds daily along with the midday meal and dinner (approximately two teaspoons with each meal). The seeds can be taken after soaking them overnight in water or in powder form as a drink in water or buttermilk 15 minutes before the meal. The powder can also be mixed with flour, rice, *dal* or vegetables.

The sugar-lowering effect of *jamun* has also been confirmed. Biochemists have isolated an active principle, alpha glucosidase inhibitor, from the fruit. This places *jamun* in the same company as the alpha glucosidase inhibitor drug, Acarbose.

The useful role of *Momordia charantia* or more simply, *karela*, however, is still suspect. However, some scientists have presented an interesting theory that it may contain a peptide which may be in the mould of vegetable insulin.

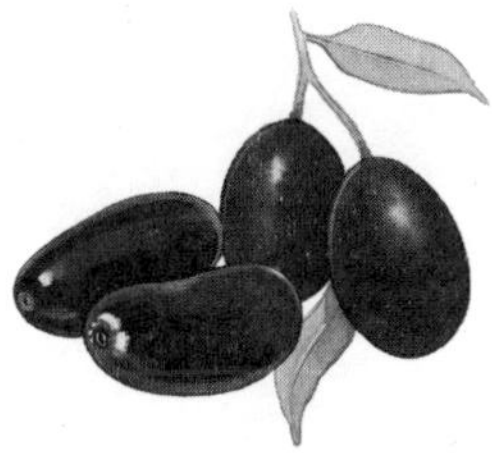

The Magic Effect

Exercise and Yoga

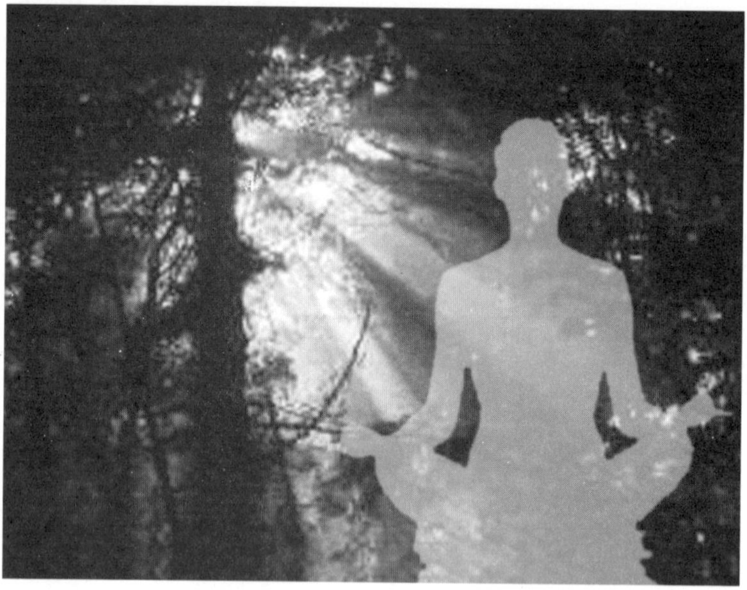

The positive role of exercise and physical activity in the management of diabetes has been emphasized in ayurveda since ancient times. In the treatise *Susruta Samhita*, written around 600 BC, Susruta has prescribed that a person with diabetes must walk at least four miles a day. Modern medicine has also ratified this advice. Research substantiates that exercise and increased physical activity bring a bounty of health benefits—especially if you have diabetes.

Every day, in every way, I am getting better and better.

Émile Coué
Formula of Autosuggestion

Benefits of exercise

By exercising regularly, you stand to gain in many ways. The benefits include:

Healthier blood sugar level: This happens because of several reasons. Each act of exercise requires energy, and this means the body uses up the excess sugar in the blood. Naturally, the body's blood sugar level falls. On top of it, the body's sensitivity to insulin improves, and this allows insulin to escort sugar into your cells, bringing a further improvement in the blood sugar level.

Reduction in weight: Regular exercise takes off pounds by burning calories and increasing your metabolism. This weight loss also helps improve the body's ability to use insulin, and thus lower the blood sugar to a healthier level.

Risk reduction in heart disease: Exercise increases the heart's pumping power, lowers the blood pressure, and improves the blood circulation. It also reduces LDL cholesterol and triglycerides which cause fat deposits in the arteries, and increases the HDL cholesterol that cleans up the arteries.

Boost to overall fitness: Exercise is a wonderful tonic for the mind and body. It heightens your mental abilities, improves your concentration and increases your creativity. It stops osteoporosis and bone loss, improves the flexibility of muscles and joints and tones up your muscles. If you exercise regularly, you feel less tired.

Reduction in stress and tension: Exercise is a balm for the mind. It eases stress, depression and negative thoughts while increasing self-esteem.

Don't you think these are good enough reasons to become active? If you feel motivated, there are a number of choices to choose from.

Exercises to choose from

Broadly, exercise is of two types: aerobic and anaerobic. Aerobic means 'with oxygen'. Such activities that require extra oxygen and whose demands can be met by increasing the breathing and heart rate, and by increased haulage of oxygen to the muscles, qualify as aerobic exercise. They benefit all people, including people with diabetes. Activities such as walking, jogging, aerobic dancing, cycling, swimming, skating, golfing, badminton and tennis are categorized under this group.

In contrast, anaerobic activities are short bursts of acute physical effort. They obtain energy from glucose metabolism which must function in the absence of oxygen. As a result, they lead to formation of lactic acid in the body. Such activities include weightlifting. People with diabetes should not perform them.

Getting started

Before getting started, it is always safe to see your doctor first. A normal examination should clear you for the fitness programme. This safeguard is a must if you are over 40.

A number of activities, including some specific yogic *asanas*, should not be done by people who have developed diabetes-related complications. For instance, *sarvanga asana* should bt strictly avoided by those with high blood pressure.

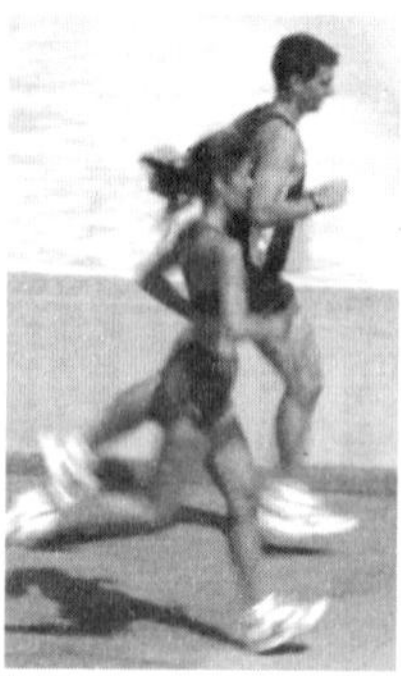

Walking is easiest

Unless you have lost the protective sensation in the feet, walking is one of the easiest ways to get aerobic exercise. It is safe and requires no special training or equipment. You just need to put on clean, smooth-fitting cotton socks, proper walking shoes, and suitable clothes for the weather before setting out. The benefit is immense: studies have established that walking for mere 30 minutes five times a week lowers insulin resistance, and improves blood sugar control.

What if you lose the sensation in your feet

Long-standing diabetes can lead to a numbness in the feet. If that happens, limit weight-bearing exercise. Repetitive exercise on insensitive feet can lead to ulceration and fractures. You must not do prolonged walking, jogging or step exercises. Rather, you may opt for swimming, cycling, chair exercises, arm exercises, and rowing. They would not exert any weight on your feet.

Draw a safe and enjoyable fitness plan

Warm up and cool down

Before you begin exercising, get your body ready. A proper warm up should include 5-10 minutes of aerobic activity at low intensity level. The warm-up session is to prepare the heart, lungs and muscles for more intense activity.

Just as at the beginning, it helps if you walk less intensely for a while to allow your heart rate to gradually slow down when you are about to finish the exercise session. A couple of slow stretches afterwards can help keep your muscles limber and prevent them from tightening up.

Do stretching exercises

Gentle stretching of the muscles should also be a part of the routine. It increases the range to which you can bend and stretch your joints, muscles and ligaments and also helps prevent joint pain and injury. Here are three stretches you can try:

Calf stretch. Stand at arm's length from the wall. Lean your upper body into the wall. Place one leg forward with knee bent. Keep your other leg back with your knee straight and your heel down. Keeping your back straight, move your hips toward the wall until you feel a stretch. Hold for 30 seconds. Relax. Repeat with the other leg. Repeat five to 10 times.

Lower back stretch. Lie on a table or bed with your hips and knees bent and your feet flat on the surface. Gently pull one knee toward your shoulder with both hands. Hold for 30 seconds. Relax. Repeat with the other leg. Repeat five to 10 times.

Chest stretch. Clasp your hands behind your head. Pull your elbows firmly back while inhaling and exhaling deeply. Hold for 30 seconds. Relax. Repeat five to 10 times.

Drink plenty of fluids

You lose fluid when you sweat, and it is important to replace this fluid. If you are not careful and get dehydrated, it can affect blood glucose level and heart function adversely. Water is the best choice. Drink plenty of it before, during and after any exercise.

How much exercise?

You should aim for at least 30 minutes of aerobic activity most days of the week. If you have not been active for a long time, start slowly and build up your endurance. Begin by exercising 10 minutes a day. Each week, increase the length of time for exercise by five minutes, until you start doing 30-45 minutes a day.

You may also break your routine into shorter intervals. You might walk for 10-15 minutes in the morning, another 10 minutes during the lunch hour, and again, for 10-15 minutes in the evening.

Listen to warning signs

Never ignore symptoms that may signal a health snag. These include:

- Dizziness or faintness
- Tightness in the chest
- Chest pain, pain in an arm or the jaw
- Palpitations
- Unexpected shortness of breath

If you experience these symptoms, talk to your doctor. Until he clears you, take a break from your fitness programme.

Yoga time

The useful role of yogic exercises (*asanas*) in lowering blood sugar has been confirmed by several researchers. The benefit extends to both the fasting and after-food blood sugar levels. Several yoga poses have been found effective. You could also try them out!

Lifting leg pose (Uttan pada asana)

Lie down on your back. Make the body straight. Keep the heels together. Bring the palms near the body on the mat. Relax and breathe freely. Stretch out the toes and make them hard and tight. Take a deep breath, and raise the legs upwards towards the sky, and gradually bring them into a perpendicular position. Hold this pose for a few seconds. Gradually increase the time to 10 seconds. While exhaling, return to the original position.

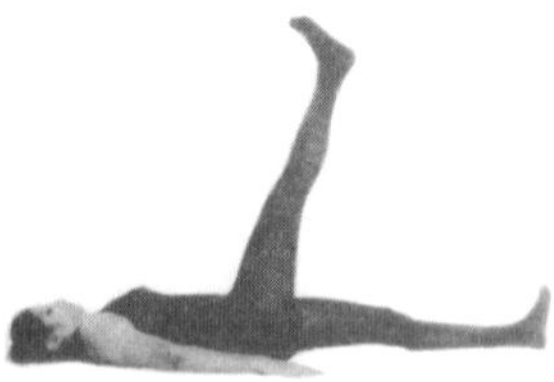

Caution: People who suffer from high blood pressure, coronary heart disease or backache should avoid this *asana*.

The serpent's pose (Bhujanga asana)

Lie down on the mat with the chest down. Keep the legs straight. Let the feet touch each other. The soles of the feet should touch face upwards. Keep the hands on two sides of the chest. Raise the head and stretch it back pushing your tongue out. Give a backward stretch to the

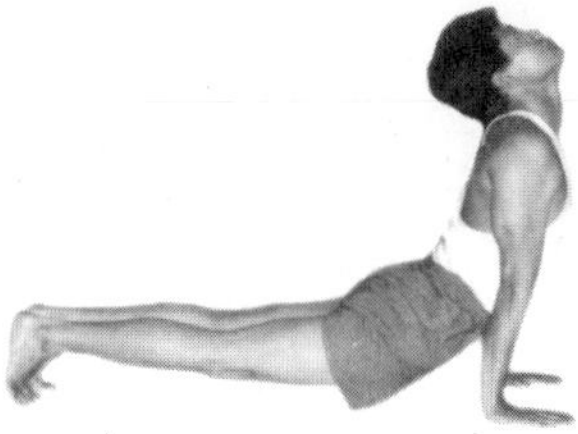

neck. Raise the chest slowly. Contract the muscles of the back. Give a backward bend to the back as much as possible. Experience a steady pull along the back from the neck downwards. After keeping the pose for a moment, lower the chest and relax the backbone. After brief relaxation, repeat the pose.

The locust pose *(Shalabh asana)*

Lie down on the mat on your stomach with chin touching the floor. Keep your hands on the side of the body, with fingers straight and touching each other. Take a deep breath, and raise your right leg slowly, without a jerk. Maintain the posture for half a minute only in the beginning and gradually increase the time. Return to your original position, relax and repeat with left leg. Next, raise both the legs together.

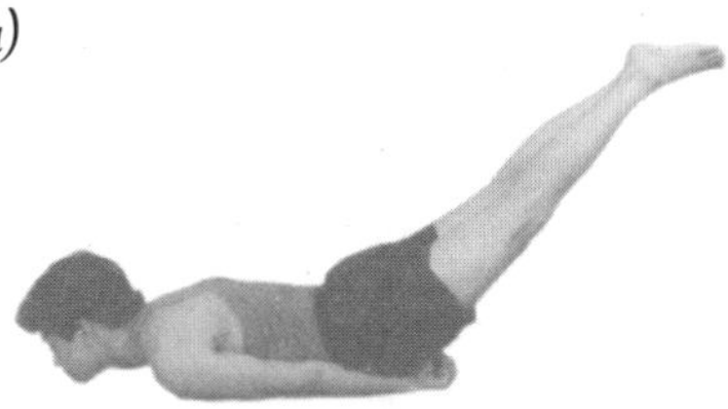

Do it two times only in the beginning, increasing gradually.

The bow pose *(Dhanur asana)*

Lie down on your stomach. Keep your arms straight on both sides. Let your chin rest on the mat. Bring the legs and heels together. Fold your legs at the knees. Bring the heels close to your hips. Grab the right ankle with your right hand, and the left with the left hand. Pull and stretch yourself upwards. Inhale, pause, exhale, pause.

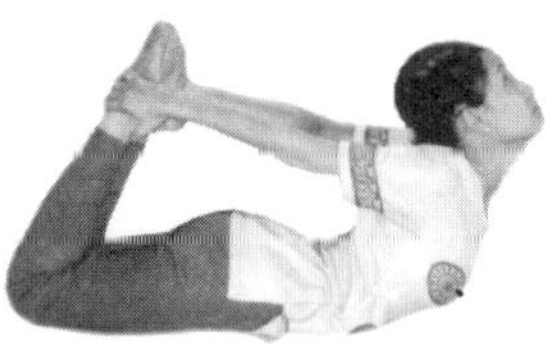

Standing on the shoulders *(Sarvanga asana)*

Lie flat on your back with the muscles relaxed. Keep the hands alongside with thighs and legs together. Slowly raise the legs. Lift the back off the ground. Prop the back with the hands. The entire weight of the body should be balanced on the shoulders and the posterior part of the neck. Maintain this pose for a few seconds to begin with. Gradually increase the time to five minutes. Return to the original position in slow motion.

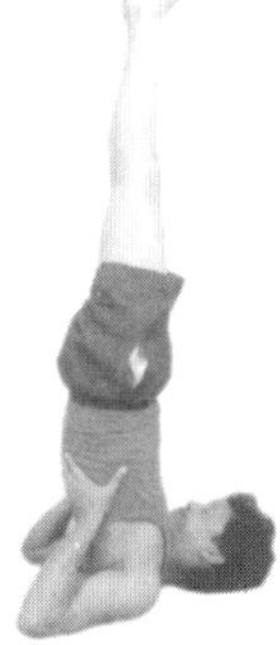

The plough pose (Hala asana)

Lie flat on the ground. Stretch out the whole body. Make yourself quite straight. Bring the heels and the toes together. Lift your toes. Throw the legs forward. Bring the thighs above your head. Your arms will rest on the floor. Hold this pose for a few minutes. Inhale as you assume the pose; exhale as you return to the normal position. Synchronize inhaling and lifting of legs.

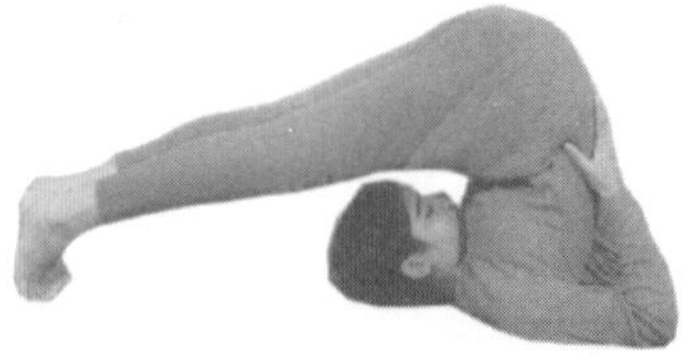

The fish pose (Matsya asana)

Sit in *padma asana* by keeping the right foot over the left thigh and the left foot over the right thigh. Lie flat on the back. Stretch the head back. The top of the head should rest firmly on the ground, and so should the buttocks, thus making a bridge of the trunk. Place your hands on the thighs. Catch your toes with your hands. When you have performed the *asana* for a few minutes, slowly release the head with the help of your hands. Sit up. Then unlock the *padma asana*.

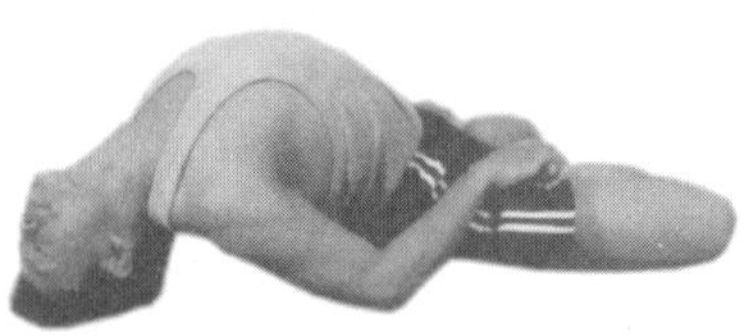

The lotus pose (Padma asana)

Sit upright. Put the right foot on the left thigh, and the left foot on the right thigh. The heels come close to each other. The hands may be placed on the knees. Keep the eyes, the neck and the head straight. Inhale, hold breath, exhale, hold breath. You may spend 1-30 minutes in this pose, and meditate.

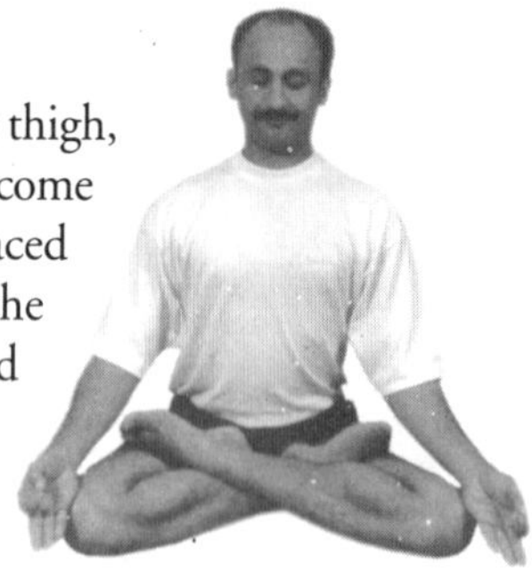

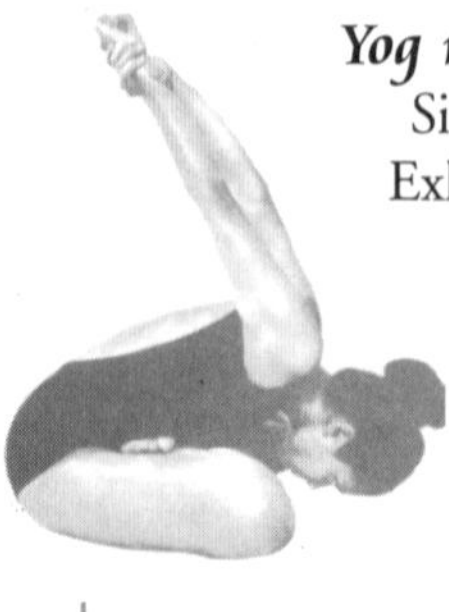

Yog mudra

Sit in the *padma asana*. Place the palms on the heels. Exhale slowly. Bend forward and touch the floor with the forehead. Return to the original position and inhale. Instead of keeping the hands on the heels, you can take them back. Catch hold of the left wrist with your right hand. Hold this pose for a few seconds.

Bending-the-back pose (Paschimottana asana)

Sit on the ground. Stretch your legs and arms stiff like a stick. Catch the toes with the thumb and index and middle fingers. While catching toes, bend the trunk forward. Exhale. Slowly bend without jerks till your forehead touches your knees. When you bend down, draw the belly back. Retain the breath till you take the forehead back to its original position. Inhale. If you find it difficult to do full *paschimottana asana*, you could begin by doing the half pose with one leg and one hand and then with the other leg and the other hand. Once the spine becomes more elastic, you can do the full pose.

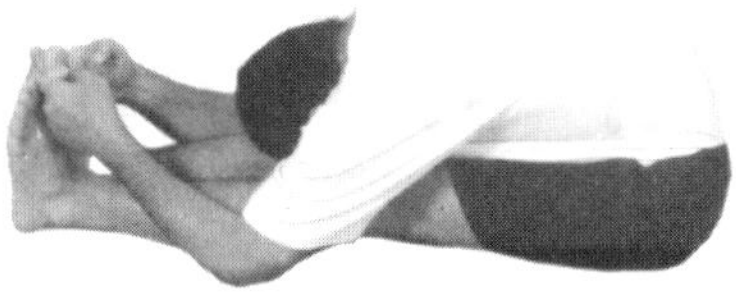

Caution: If you suffer from sciatica or bad joints, avoid doing this *asana*.

Pranayama

Pranayama is the yoga of breathing. It has three stages: exhalation, inhalation, and retention of breath. The technique is simple. Sit on the ground in a lotus or easy pose. Hold the spine, neck and head absolutely upright. Look straight. Stretch your arms and rest your wrists on the knees. Bring your thumb and index finger in apposition so that they form a circle. Keep the other three fingers straight. Breathe normally.

Now, exhale slowly through both the nostrils and at the same time, contract your abdominal muscles to expel air from the lungs. Pause for a second. Next, inhale as deep as you can, sucking in air through the nose, and letting it fill all the vessels in the body. The abdominal muscles should also expand this time. Pause for a second. Repeat exhalation. Continue the same process ten or fifteen times.

after-meal glucose. They work best for people in whom the disease is less than five-years old, and who still can produce some insulin on their own. Often the first choice, especially in overweight people, sulfonylureas are initiated at low doses and increased at one-to two-week intervals, based on the individual blood glucose levels.

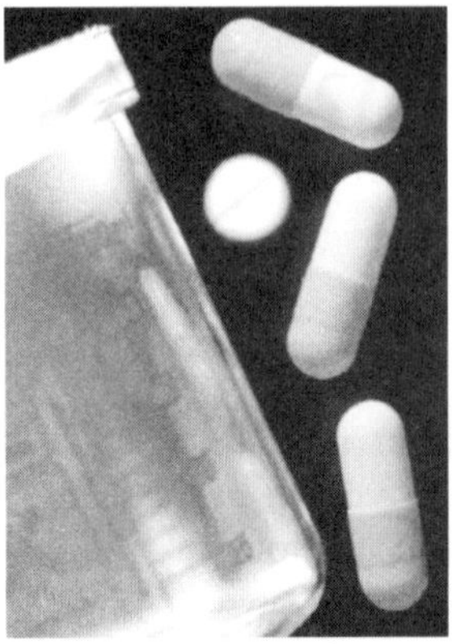

Though Tolbutamide, Chlorpropamide and Glibenclamide, the first generation sulfonylureas, may evoke nostalgia in the older people, they have now largely been replaced by the second-generation pills: Glipizide, Gliclazide and Glimepiride. These newer drugs are preferred over their forerunners since they are less likely to cause low blood sugar (hypoglycaemia), and do not linger for long in your circulatory system, thus reducing the risk of complications.

Possible side effects: Low blood sugar is the most common side effect of sulfonylureas, especially during the initial months of therapy. This risk is much greater if liver or kidneys are not functioning well. There's also the risk of weight gain, a side effect against which you should be careful.

Safeguards: Never exercise more than usual or skip a meal after you have taken a sulfonylurea, as it can lead to an unusually low blood sugar. Alcohol and some drugs, including decongestants, can also cause this problem. Conversely, some medications such as steroids, beta-blockers, and niacin decrease the effectiveness of sulfonylureas. Hence, before taking another medication you should always check with the doctor.

Meglitinides

Chemically different from sulfonylureas, meglitinides act by a similar mechanism. Repaglinide is the only drug available in this class. It causes a rapid, but short-lived release of insulin by the pancreas. Because it works quickly and its effects diminish rapidly, it is taken with meals. It kicks into action shortly thereafter, when your blood sugar level is highest.

Biguanides

Metformin and Phenformin are members of the biguanide family. They reduce the amount of sugar the liver releases into the bloodstream and also improve the body's response to insulin. They reduce fasting blood glucose, lower cholesterol and triglycerides, and promote a modest weight loss. For this reason, people with type 2 diabetes who are overweight are often prescribed a biguanide.

Possible side effects: In some people, Metformin might cause an unpleasant metallic taste in the mouth, loss of appetite, nausea, abdominal bloating, gas or diarrhoea. These effects usually occur during the first few weeks of treatment but decrease with time.

A rare but serious side effect of Metformin is lactic acidosis—a build-up of lactic acid in your body. If you have a kidney disease, congestive heart failure or any other disease that may cause your body to produce too much lactic acid, you should avoid the drug.

Safeguards: Since Metformin and alcohol do not mix well, it is better not to take alcohol. It is also important to stop taking Metformin prior to undergoing any imaging procedure involving the use of an intravenous dye. Such procedures include intravenous pyelography (IVP), angiography, computed tomography (CT) scan and a host of other X-ray studies.

Alpha-glucosidase inhibitors

Alpha-glucosidase inhibitors—Acarbose and Miglitol—taken just before each meal, block the action of enzyme that breaks down carbohydrates into simple sugar in the intestinal lumen. As a result, sugar is absorbed into the bloodstream more slowly than usual, and this limits the rapid rise in blood sugar that usually occurs right after a meal.

Possible side effects: Alpha-glucosidase inhibitors often cause bothersome side effects, including abdominal bloating or discomfort, gas, and diarrhoea. Doctors get round the problem by starting you with a low dose of medication and then gradually stepping it up.

Safeguards: You should not take Acarbose or Miglitol if you suffer from an inflammatory bowel disease, poor gastric function, or kidney disease. You must also avoid the use of antacids.

Thiazolidinediones

A new class of medications, Pioglitazone and Rosiglitazone help reduce the fasting blood sugar by making your body tissues more sensitive to insulin. The more effective insulin is at escorting sugar from the blood into your cells, the less sugar remains in your bloodstream. These drugs also help lower the amount of triglycerides in the blood.

Possible side effects: Side effects from the medications may include swelling, weight gain and fatigue. You also have to be vigilant about the rare side effect of liver injury. Your doctor might ask you to undergo blood tests to assess the health of your liver before starting on a thiazolidinedione, and then every two months during the first year of therapy.

Safeguards: Thiazolidinediones can induce ovulation in women. If you are taking birth control pills, they may make the contraceptives less effective.

Combination therapy

By combining medications from different drug classes, which work in different ways, the glucose-lowering effects of diabetes medications can be maximized. The most common combination therapy uses a sulfonylurea and Metformin, but a sulfonylurea can equally be combined with Acarbose or Miglitol, or Pioglitazone or Rosiglitazone. Likewise, Metformin gels well with Acarbose, Rosiglitazone or Pioglitazone. Oral diabetes medications can also usefully be combined with insulin in moments of need.

Insulin

Until 1922, when insulin first became commercially available to the public, people diagnosed with diabetes faced a bleak future. Treatments were severe—some people were purposely starved so that their blood sugar levels could be controlled, while others were given enormous amounts of fluid, even alcohol, to flush their system of impurities. Regardless of the treatment, most people did not live longer than a year after their diagnosis. The landmark discovery of insulin in 1921 changed this all. Today, it offers a new lease of life to people with type 1 diabetes, but it is also an effective medication for treating type 2 diabetes, at the time when everything else fails.

Sources of insulin

Nowadays, the most widely used form of insulin is synthetic human insulin. It is called human insulin because its chemical makeup is identical to that of insulin produced by the human pancreas; but this insulin is produced in laboratories with the help of special genetically engineered bacteria which churn it out in large amounts.

Before this advancement, the insulin used to treat diabetes exclusively came from the pancreases of cattle (bovine insulin) or pigs (porcine insulin). For decades researchers worked to improve the purity of insulin and to develop insulin preparations with longer-lasting action in the body. However, animal insulin was never free from limitations. Some people suffered allergic reactions because of protein impurities, while others experienced skin irritation at the site of the injection. For these reasons, animal insulin is used less commonly now, but being cheaper than human insulin, it continues to be of use, particularly in the developing countries.

Why only shots

Insulin is always administered by injection, using a syringe, an insulin pen, or an insulin pump. It is not available in pill form because it gets destroyed in the stomach during digestion, and cannot enter the bloodstream.

Types of insulin

Many types of insulin are used, and they differ in the time it takes for them to begin working and in the period for which they are effective.

Regular insulin

Regular insulin is clear or crystalline in appearance. It starts working quickly, by 30 minutes to one hour, working its hardest between three to four hours, and its action lasts for six hours.

NPH and lente insulin

NPH and lente insulin are a cloudy suspension. They start working later than short-acting insulin, and their effect lasts longer. They start working by two hours; work hardest between eight to 12 hours, and their effect lasts for 24 hours.

Pre-mixed insulin

To suit different people's needs, pre-mixed insulin with varying proportions of regular and lente insulin, and other short- and intermediate-acting insulin are also available commercially. They usually start working in 30 minutes to one hour, peak in their action in three hours and again at eight to 12 hours, and continue to work for 24 hours.

Ultralente insulin

A long-acting insulin, Ultralente insulin is a cloudy suspension. It takes several hours to work, but the duration of its peak action is greater than that of other forms of insulin. It starts working by seven hours, is effective for more than 22 hours, and its action lasts for up to 36 hours.

Insulin regimens

The type and dosage of insulin a person needs, depends on the pattern of the disease. You may need one or two types of insulin on a daily basis.

Mixing two types of insulin can mimic natural insulin production in the body more accurately. You might take a short-acting insulin to simulate insulin secretion at mealtime and a longer-acting insulin to mimic basal insulin secretions. Your doctor will guide you in deciding the insulin regimen which will work best for you. Several types of insulin regimens exist:

Mixed dose. You inject both short-acting and intermediate-acting insulins — mixed in one syringe — each morning.

Premixed single dose. You inject a dose of premixed insulin each morning.

Split dose. You give yourself two injections of intermediate-acting insulin each day. These injections are usually given before breakfast and before the evening meal, or before breakfast and at bedtime.

Split mixed dose. You give yourself two injections that contain a combination of a short-acting and an intermediate-acting insulin — mixed in one syringe — each day. These are generally given before breakfast and before the evening meal.

Split premixed dose. You give yourself two injections of premixed insulin daily. These are usually given before breakfast and before the evening meal, or before breakfast and at bedtime.

Using insulin

When first diagnosed with diabetes, you may feel frightened or nervous about injecting yourself with insulin. That's natural. Learning about the process and doing it a few times will help you feel more comfortable.

Select the site

It is safe to inject insulin into any area of the body where a layer of fatty tissue is present and where large blood vessels, nerves, muscles and bones do not course close to the surface. However, since insulin is absorbed most evenly from the abdomen, except for the 2-inch area around the navel, it is best to administer insulin in the abdomen. Rotate the site of each injection each time. You may also use other areas for injection, such as your hips, buttocks, upper arms and thighs. After you determine the site for your insulin injection, clean it with an alcohol swab, and allow it to dry before giving yourself an injection.

Prepare well

Collect the materials you will need: alcohol swab, insulin and the syringe. Check the insulin bottle for any changes in the insulin. Make sure no clumping, precipitation or change in clarity or colour has occurred. Any change in appearance may mean that the insulin has lost its potency. Now, wash your hands with soap and water.

How to draw insulin

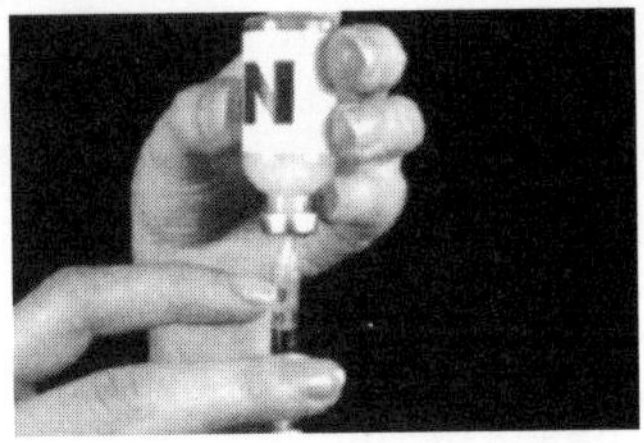

With time and practice, drawing insulin into the syringe becomes routine. Here's how to do it: Gently roll the bottle of insulin between your hands to mix the insulin. Shaking it may decrease its potency. Wipe off the top of the insulin bottle with an alcohol wipe. Remove the needle cap from the syringe. Pull the plunger to draw into the syringe an amount of air equal to the amount of insulin you need. Insert the needle through the rubber stopper of the insulin bottle and push the air in the syringe into the bottle. While keeping the needle in the bottle, turn the bottle completely upside down. Pull the plunger on the syringe slightly past the number of units of insulin you are to inject. Be sure that you are withdrawing insulin, not air. Air is not dangerous but it can decrease the amount of insulin in the syringe. Remove air bubbles either by pushing the insulin back into the bottle and withdrawing it again or snapping the syringe sharply with your finger and then pushing the plunger to expel the air into the bottle. Check the amount of insulin in the syringe. Pull the needle out of the bottle.

How to inject insulin

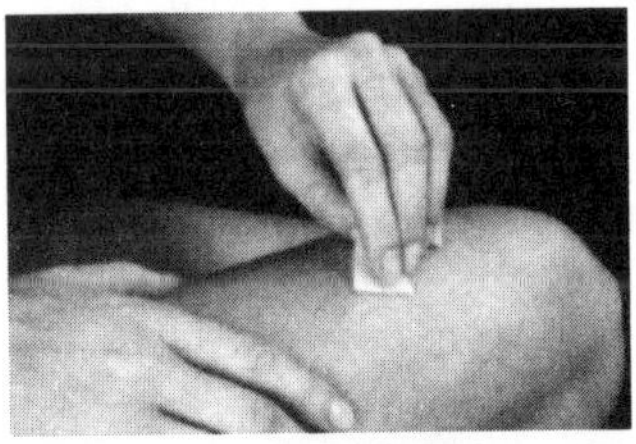

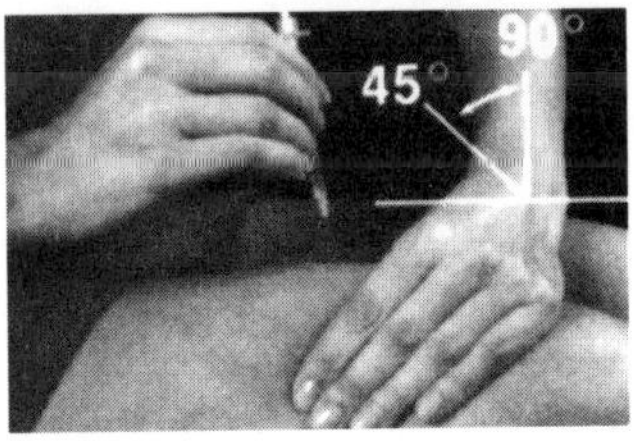

Now, it is time to inject the insulin. Hold the syringe like a pencil. Quickly insert the entire length of the needle into a fold of your skin at a 90-degree angle. If you are thin, it may be best to inject at a 45-degree angle. Release the pinched skin and inject the insulin by gently pushing the plunger all the way down at a steady, moderate rate. Place the alcohol swab on your skin next to the needle and withdraw the needle. Apply gentle pressure with the alcohol swab at the injection site for three to five seconds. Don't rub.

Minimize skin reactions, pain and bumps

Occasionally, especially when you first start using insulin, you may notice redness and slight swelling at the injection site. This irritation usually disappears in two to three weeks. To avoid this, let the injection site dry after cleaning it with alcohol. If the skin irritation lasts more than two to three weeks or causes you discomfort, talk to your doctor.

To minimize pain during injections, make sure the insulin is at room temperature. If it is too cold, it can cause pain. Relax your muscles in the area of the injection, and be quick in penetrating the skin with the needle.

Some people develop indentations, hard lumps or thickened skin in areas where they inject insulin. You can avoid this problem by rotating the site of your injections well.

Insulin pens

Insulin pens are extremely innovative. They are a convenient, accurate and discreet means of receiving insulin. The device looks like a pen with a cartridge—but the cartridge is filled with insulin rather than ink. Some pens use disposable cartridges containing pre-filled insulin. Other pens are completely disposable. You place a fine point needle on the tip of the pen, turn a dial to select the desired insulin dose, insert the needle under your skin and then click down on a button at the end of the pen to deliver the insulin. The pen can be easily transported in a purse, briefcase or a coat's long pocket.

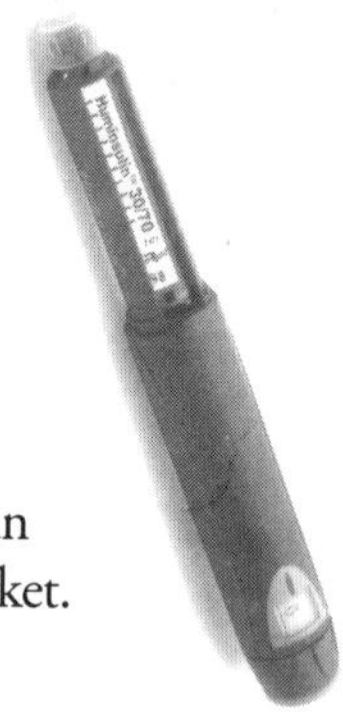

Insulin pumps

Today, portable insulin pumps are also available. They provide a continuous supply of insulin, and eliminate the need for daily shots. Smaller than a deck of cards, they can be hooked to a belt. Essentially, a small pumping device that you wear outside your body, an insulin pump contains a syringe reservoir that you fill with insulin. A small, flexible tube connects the reservoir of insulin to a catheter that is inserted under the skin of your abdomen. The pump disperses the desired amount of insulin through the catheter into your body continuously by slow infusion. You can also programme it to deliver larger amounts of insulin during meals. Every second or third day you need to change the infusion site. To do this, you pull out the catheter and insert a new one at a different site. The reservoir that holds the insulin also needs to be refilled every few days.

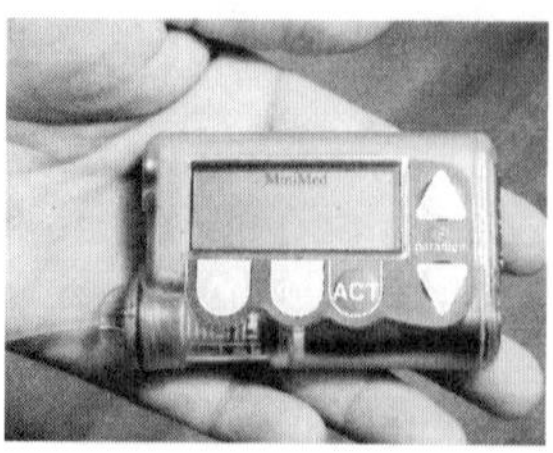

The main advantage of the insulin pump is improved blood sugar control. The pump enables you to match better your insulin needs and insulin delivery. However, its use is not for everybody. It is expensive and needs some basic understanding and training, before yor can use it well.

The possibility of insulin sprays

For the last several years, bio scientists have been working hard at developing alternative ways to deliver insulin. Efforts are afoot to develop a special form of insulin that could be taken as a spray. Two types of inhaled insulin preparations are currently under experimentation. While one is deliverable through the mouth, the other could be received through the nose. However, it may still be several years, before researchers can perfect this new form of insulin and check whether it would be as effective and reliable as the currently available one.

Reduce Your Risk of Complications

Self-Care

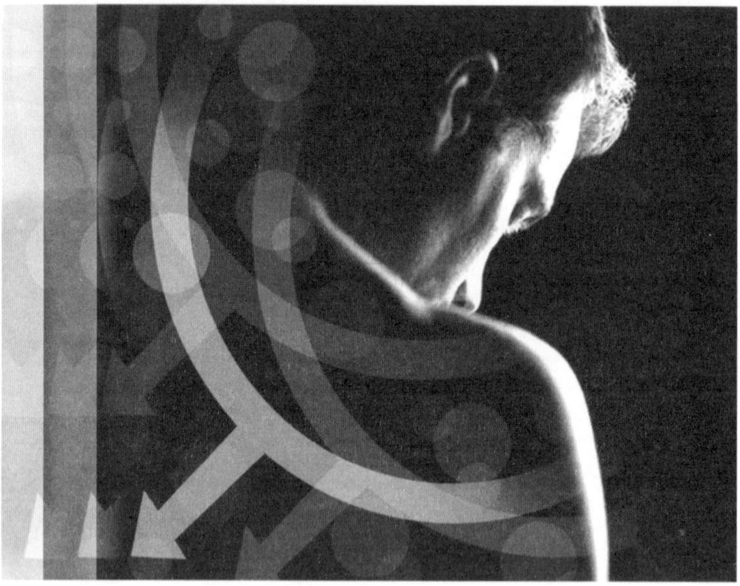

A healthy body and mind are the greatest treasures a man can have. Yet, once diabetes makes its foray, a threat looms large. The disease can impinge on your well-being by adversely affecting vital organs such as the eyes, gums, heart and circulatory system, kidneys, and nerves. Your chances of complications such as coronary heart disease, high blood pressure, stroke, partial loss of vision, kidney failure, and nerve damage rise. However, a stitch in time can still save nine. A better regulated blood sugar and sensible self-care can restrict the damage and uphold the joy of life.

Life is real! Life is earnest!
And the grave is not its goal.

H W Longfellow
A Psalm of Life

Go for an annual medical check-up

Beyond the regular follow-up visits to your diabetes doctor, you must undergo a thorough medical check-up once a year. This will facilitate an early diagnosis of any emerging problem that diabetes may cause. You would be required to take screening tests for a variety of conditions, such as kidney, heart or circulatory problems. Should there be any signs of a disease or complication, taking timely action may still limit the damage.

Have a regular eye check-up

Diabetes can affect the eyes adversely. A fluctuant blood sugar can alter the thickness of the natural lens and thus influence the focussing power of the eye. Or it might lead to more serious damage by promoting growth of frail new blood vessels in the retina that leak from time to time and disrupt vision. Diabetes might also lead to rise in internal eye pressure, a condition called glaucoma, or spur premature clouding of lens, causing cataract.

Regular eye check-ups with an eye doctor can detect the signs of possible complications while they are most amenable to treatment. The following eye tests done once a year may be of use:

Visual acuity test: This test measures the sharpness of your vision. The eye doctor or optometrist will check how well you read letters from across the room. Your eyes will be tested one at a time, while the other eye is covered. At the same sitting, you might also be tested on how well you can read the close-up letters by using a specially designed card.

Visual field charting (perimetry): This test assesses how much area you can see in front of you without moving your eyes. In a computerized

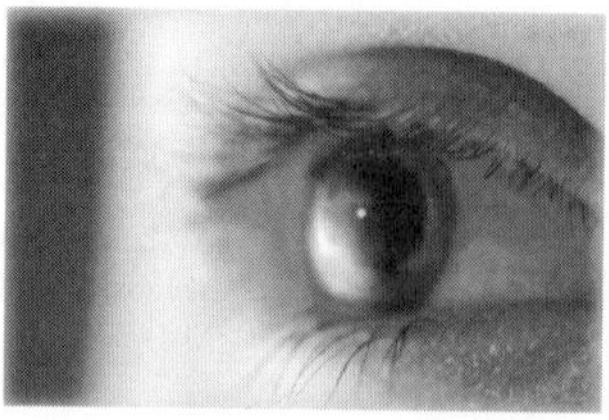

perimetry test, you look at a testing screen on which a machine flashes spots of light. The flashes will be at different locations on the screen and of varying brightness. Your job is to press a button each time you see a flash. The machine records your responses and maps the areas where vision is good.

Retinal examination: During a retinal examination, the eye doctor puts dilating drops in your eyes to open your pupils wide and provide a bigger window to the back of your eye. Then, by using an ophthalmoscope, he can diagnose abnormalities in the vitreous, the retina, the optic nerve and the vascular coat of the eye. This test is especially important because retinal damage is the most common eye complication in diabetes. Treatment with laser can restrict the damage.

Slit-lamp examination: A slit lamp allows the doctor to see the different structures at the front of your eye — cornea, iris and lens and the anterior chamber — in cross-section and under magnification. Since diabetes is known to spur early cataract, this examination can pick the changes in the lens early.

Glaucoma test (tonometry): By measuring the internal pressure of your eye, the eye doctor can determine whether you are developing glaucoma. The disease can gradually narrow your field of vision and produce tube vision and blindness.

Fluorescein angiography: Fluorescein angiography is a special diagnostic test used for evaluating diseases of the retina and the vascular coat (choroid) of the eye. To carry out the test, fluorescein (a dye) is injected in your arm vein. As it circulates through your eye, the blood vessels in your retina and choroid stand out as bright yellow. A camera takes flash pictures every few seconds for several minutes. This test may not be necessary every year, but it can be very useful in assessing the damage to the normal eye blood vessels and also view the abnormal blood vessels that might arise in your retina.

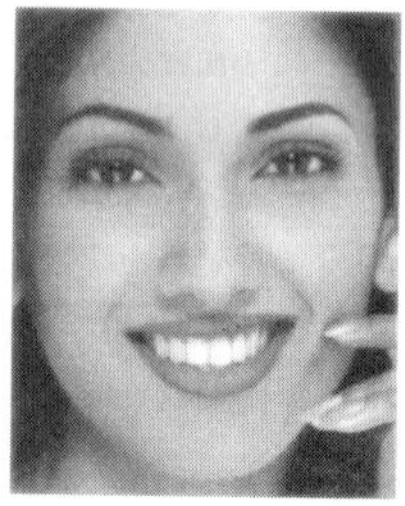

Protect against gum disease

High blood sugar can cause infection and inflammation in your gums. You may develop pyorrhoea—a gum disease that can cause bad breath, bleeding from the gums, and loosen out your teeth. To help prevent damage to your gums and teeth:

- ♥ Brush your teeth twice a day.
- ♥ Rinse your mouth after each meal.
- ♥ See your dentist every six months.
- ♥ Look for early signs of gum disease, such as bleeding gums, redness and swelling. If you notice them, see your dentist.

Safeguard your heart and circulatory system

If you have diabetes, you are twice as likely to develop high blood pressure as individuals with normal blood sugar. Your risk of a heart attack, stroke or other circulatory problems is also huge. However, you can fight these odds by monitoring your blood pressure, managing your cholesterol, taking a tablet of aspirin daily and not smoking.

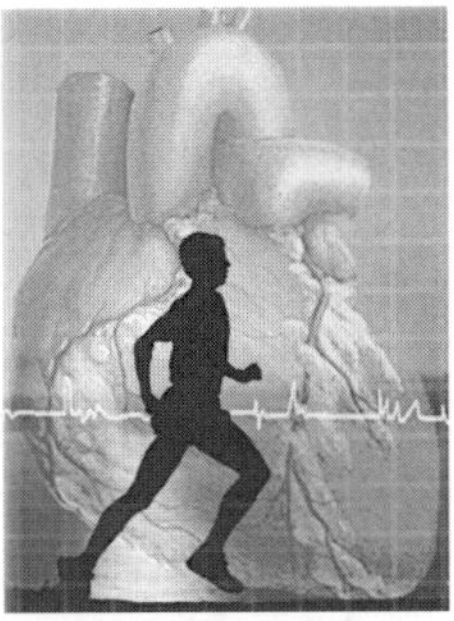

Monitor your blood pressure: Adults with diabetes must keep their blood pressure below 130/80 points. The same lifestyle changes that can improve your blood sugar — a balanced diet, regular exercise and reduction in weight — can help reduce your blood pressure. Limiting salt (sodium) intake and alcohol is also most useful.

If this does not check your blood pressure, your doctor may prescribe blood pressure-lowering medication. The drugs most commonly used for people with diabetes are angiotensin-converting enzyme (ACE) inhibitors like Lisinopril or Enlapril; and angiotensin II receptor blockers like Losartan. These medications have a low rate of side effects, and they help protect your kidneys and heart, which are at high risk of damage from both diseases. Other high blood pressure medications prescribed to people with diabetes include diuretics, beta-blockers, and calcium channel-blocker drugs.

Tidy up your lipid numbers: People with diabetes often have wonky lipid numbers that contribute to higher rates of coronary heart disease and other circulatory problems. The goal should be to tidy up these numbers: lower your LDL cholesterol to less than 100 mg/dl; decrease triglycerides to less than 150 mg/dl; and raise the HDL cholesterol to more than 40 mg/dl.

Healthful changes in diet, including restriction of saturated fats to less than 10 per cent of the total daily calories, increasing the natural fibre content by taking more of natural foods and less of processed and junk foods, and limiting daily calories are the first prerequisites. Regular exercise can also help bring an improvement. If these measures do not suffice, your doctor may prescribe you a statin such as Atorvastatin.

Take an aspirin daily: When you have diabetes, the platelet cells tend to be stickier, and you are at an increased risk of formation of blood clots. Aspirin is an anti-clotting, anti-platelet drug that decreases the stickiness of the platelets, and reduces the risks of heart attack and stroke.

Unless there is good reason not to take it, you should be taking an aspirin every day. It can reduce your risk of heart attack by up to 60 per cent. The recommended dose is anywhere from 75 mg a day, the amount found in a baby aspirin, to 325 mg a day, the amount in an adult tablet.

You should not, however, take aspirin if you have allergy to aspirin or suffer from peptic ulcer, liver disease or gout.

Do not smoke: If you have diabetes and you smoke, you are three times more likely than non-smokers with diabetes to die of heart disease or stroke, and you are more likely to develop circulation problems in your feet. Therefore, unless you wish to commit hara-kiri, you may as well stop smoking now.

Look after your feet

Diabetes can damage the nerves and reduce blood flow to your feet. Once the nerves are damaged, you lose the protective sensation. You may develop a blister or cut your foot and not realize it. If the blood flow is reduced, the feet receive less blood to nourish the tissues, and it is harder for cuts and sores to heal. A seemingly small and insignificant injury can quickly progress into a larger problem.

However, if you observe regular preventive care, you can protect your feet:

♥ Wash your feet each day with lukewarm water.

♥ Wash your feet with a gentle, massage-like motion, using a soft washcloth or sponge and a mild soap. Dry your skin by blotting or patting. Do not rub because you may rub too hard and accidentally damage your skin. Dry carefully between your toes to help prevent fungal infection.

♥ Moisturize your skin. Diabetes could leave your skin dry. Since dry skin can itch and crack, and can easily get infected, protect against dry skin by using a moisturizer regularly.

♥ Trim your toenails carefully. Bathe your feet in warm water and clean your toes carefully using a soft toothbrush and mild soap. Then cut the nails straight across so that they are even with the end of your toe. File rough edges. Be especially careful not to injure the surrounding skin. If you notice redness around the nails, report this to your doctor.

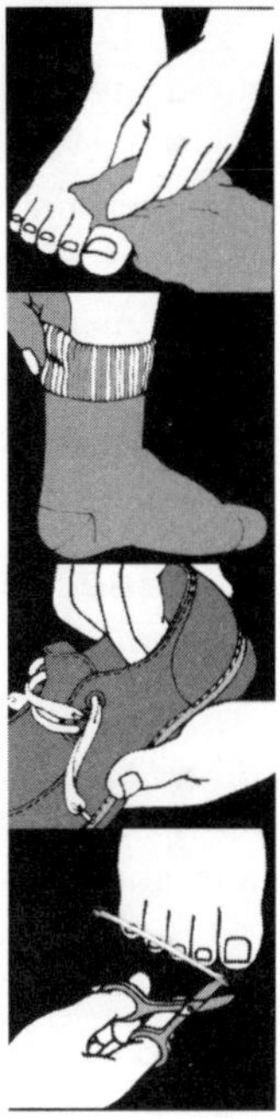

♥ Wear clean, dry socks, preferably cotton-made. Avoid those with tight elastic bands that reduce circulation.

♥ Protect your feet by wearing shoes, or sturdy slippers. Look inside your shoes for tears or rough edges that might injure your feet. Shake out your shoes before you put them on to make sure nothing is inside, such as a pebble. Always select a comfortable pair of footwear, that isn't narrow, allows air to circulate, is low-heeled, and has a flexible sole.

♥ If your feet lose sensation, be vigilant. Take care that you do not burn them by keeping them too close to a heater during the winter months.

♥ Do not use a file or scissors on calluses, corns or bunions. You can injure your feet that way. Also, do not put chemicals on your feet, such as wart removing plasters. Instead, see your doctor.

♥ Check your feet every day. Look for blisters, cuts, bruises, cracks, peeling, redness, and swelling.

♥ Do not delay treatment. If a wound isn't healing, appears to be getting bigger or looks as if it may be in-fected, see your doctor.

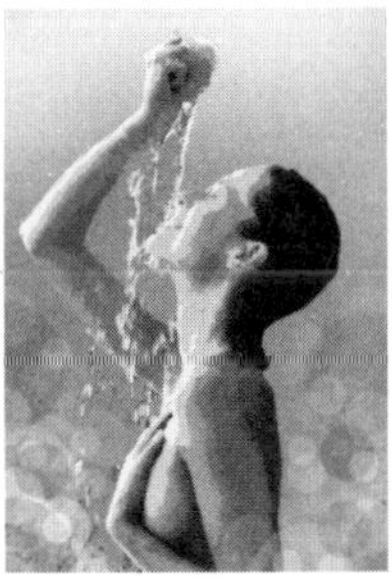

Skin care

♥ Maintain good hygiene. Take a shower every day. Use a mild soap, and clean yourself. Dry your skin by blotting or patting with a soft towel. Do not leave any wet areas because that can encourage fungal growth.

♥ Apply talcum powder on such areas of the body which sweat more like the armpits, inner folds of upper thighs, and the area below the breasts.

♥ Never wear underpants that are tight around the thighs. Also, avoid tights, skin-hugging jeans and nylons. Instead, prefer loose-fit cottons.

Travel safety

♥ Prepare well. Carry medical identification with you and bring enough diabetes supplies and medications to last the entire trip — plus a little extra in case of scheduling changes. Do not put these items in checked bags. Keep them in your carry-on bag.

♥ Take along food such as biscuits, glucose or candies to treat low blood sugar or in case you do not eat on schedule.

♥ Never take a pair of new shoes with you. Try them out on the home terrain, before using them for travel. It is also a good idea to pack two pairs of good walking shoes.

♥ As much as possible, try to follow your daily walking and eating regimen.

♥ Find out how to say in the native tongue, 'I am a diabetic. I need to see a doctor'. It can save the day in a moment of crisis.

Diabetes-related emergencies

Low blood sugar (hypoglycaemia)

This emergency can occur when too little food, excess medication, or excess exercise causes a sudden lowering of sugar level in the blood. Unless treated rightly and timely, it may cause seizures or loss of consciousness, and may even prove fatal.

Symptoms of low blood sugar include sudden weakness, irritability, sweating, trembling, shakiness, and headache followed by double vision, dizziness and confusion. The person may also behave irrationally, and may become unusually aggressive.

If you feel that you may be having this problem, try eating something containing sugar, such as glucose biscuits, sugar cubes, or candy. A drink containing glucose or fruit juice would also serve the purpose equally well. If a glucometer is handy, check your blood sugar level.

If you are helping someone in this condition, seek emergency medical attention if the person does not benefit with something containing sugar. If symptoms persist beyond 30 minutes after the home treatment, take him or her to a doctor. Remain with the person for the next one hour after recovery to ensure that he or she is thinking clearly.

Diabetic ketoacidosis

This complication occurs when the blood sugar level happens to be too high and the body's chemistry becomes severely deranged. This complication usually occurs in persons with type 1 diabetes who are very ill or neglect their insulin treatment. It can also sometimes be the first symptom of previously undiagnosed diabetes. Nausea, vomiting, abdominal pain, weakness, thirst, sweet-smelling acidotic breath and deeper and more rapid breathing — all can precede gradual confusion and loss of consciousness. The condition demands immediate attention under admittance to a medical facility.

●●●